GENTLE YOGA

OSTEOPOROSIS

Featuring Contributions By

LAURIE SANFORD

D0954960

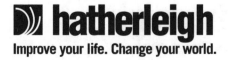

hatherleigh
Improve your life. Change your world.

Gentle Yoga for Osteoporosis

Hatherleigh Press is committed to preserving and protecting the natural resources of the Earth. Environmentally responsible and sustainable practices are embraced within the company's mission statement. Hatherleigh Press is a member of the Publishers Earth Alliance, committed to preserving and protecting the natural resources of the planet while developing a sustainable business model for the book publishing industry.

This book was edited and designed in the village of Hobart, New York. Hobart is a community that has embraced books and publishing as a component of its livelihood. There are several unique bookstores in the village. For more information, please visit www.hobartbookvillage.com.

Library of Congress Cataloging-in-Publication Data is available.
ISBN: 978-1-57826-397-4

Disclaimer: Consult your physician before beginning any exercise program. The author and publisher of this book and workout disclaim any liability, personal or professional, resulting from the misapplication of any of the following procedures described in this publication.

Cover Design by Heather Daugherty
Interior Design by Heather White
Photography by Catarina Astrom

10 9 8 7 6 5 4 3 2 1

Printed in the United States

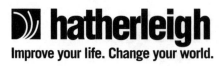

Improve your life. Change your world.

www.hatherleighpress.com

TABLE OF CONTENTS

ACKNOWLEDGMENTS

Hatherleigh Press would like to extend a special thank you to Jo Brielyn—without your hard work and dedication this book would not have been possible.

CHAPTER 1

WHAT IS OSTEOPOROSIS?

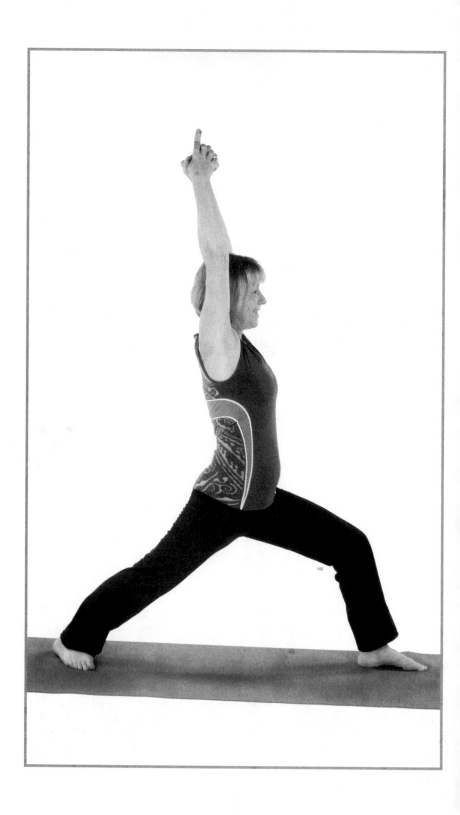

O steoporosis is a disease that causes the bones to lose density or mass. The name derives from its literal meaning, which is "porous bone". Osteoporosis is a serious condition because as the bones become less dense, they also become weaker and the risk of fracture increases. Healthy bones that are viewed under a microscope resemble a honeycomb. Examination of a similar section of bone in a person with osteoporosis will reveal much larger spaces and holes in the honeycomb. It is those expanding spaces that make the bones more fragile and prone to breakage. Bones that are affected by osteoporosis often break from injuries that would not normally cause a bone to fracture. The breaks related to osteoporosis usually happen from minor falls and can even be caused by seemingly harmless actions like sneezing, coughing, or bumping into something. Loss of bone is gradual and usually pain free, and there are no signs to indicate the development of the disease. Due to the lack of symptoms, many people do not discover they have osteoporosis until the first painful fracture takes place. That is why osteoporosis is referred to as a "silent disease".

The most common breaks related to osteoporosis happen to the spine, hip, and wrist. Fractures of the spine (also known as vertebral fractures) and hip are cause for special concern because they can lead to considerable pain and damage (like loss of height and deformity of the spine). They may also require painful surgery or the loss of mobility and independent living. The frequency of these fractures, especially those of the spine and hip, increases in both women and men as they grow older. Fortunately, people with osteoporosis or osteopenia (thinning of the bones) can prevent many fractures by adopting the right combination of lifestyle changes and medical treatment.

Who Gets Osteoporosis and What Causes It?

The National Osteoporosis Foundation estimates that about 10 million Americans already have osteoporosis and another 34 million have low bone density (called osteopenia), which places them at high risk for osteoporosis and broken bones. That means the disease affects about 55% of the people in the United States aged 50 or older. While osteoporosis can affect both men and women at any age, the disease is most common among older women. In fact, of the 10 million Americans currently diagnosed with osteoporosis, 8 million are female.

The amount of bone mass a person gains during youth is directly related to his or her risk of developing osteoporosis later in life. The greater his or her peak bone mass, the lower the risk. After the body reaches its peak bone mass, it maintains the bone strength through a process known as remodeling. Bones are remodeled when the old bone is removed (resorption) and new bone is created to take its place (formation). During youth and young adulthood, bone formation generally takes place quicker than bone resorption. In later years, resorption happens at a faster rate than new bone can be formed, and bone loss results. The presence of factors that speed up bone remodeling will also lead to a more rapid loss of bone mass and bones that are more easily fractured.

There are many factors that lead to bone loss and osteoporosis, some that can be changed and others that cannot. Awareness of these risk factors is important to the prevention, early diagnosis, and treatment of osteoporosis.

Common fixed risk factors for osteoporosis include:

Age: People of any age can get osteoporosis, but the risk increases with age. It is more common in individuals over the age of 50.

Gender: Women develop osteoporosis more often than men because they begin with a lower bone density and are also more susceptible to bone loss as they age. Women—especially those who are post-menopausal or whose ovaries have been removed—are at an even greater risk because their bodies produce less estrogen, which is a hormone that increases the thickness of bones and slows bone loss.

Family history: Genetics and heredity play a major role in bone loss, osteoporosis, and fractures. A history of bone fractures with an individual's parents or immediate family members increases his or her risk of fracturing bones and developing osteoporosis.

History of prior fractures: A person who has suffered a previous fracture is 86% more likely to have another fracture than someone with no prior fractures.

Ethnicity: Caucasian and Asian women are at the highest risk for osteoporosis. Fewer incidences are reported among African-American and Hispanic ethnic groups, but there is still a significant risk present.

Body size: Small, thin women are at greater risk for developing osteoporosis.

Low estrogen (for women), low testosterone (for men), and imbalances in other hormones (such as growth hormones): Deficiencies of all these hormones negatively affect bone density.

Other preexisting conditions that directly or indirectly affect the body's ability to replace lost bone tissue (called bone remodeling) or influence mobility and balance: These diseases and conditions take a heavy toll on bones and make an individual more susceptible to fractures and osteoporosis. A few examples are rheumatoid arthritis, nutritional and gastrointestinal problems (like Crohn's disease), endocrine disorders (such as diabetes or hyperparathyroidism), hematological disorders/malignancies, asthma, and immobility.

Use of some prescription drugs and medical treatments: There are side effects linked to some medications that cause bones to become weaker or increase the likelihood of falling, which in turn may lead to a greater risk of fractures or osteoporosis. These medications include glucocorticoid therapy, certain immunosuppressants, lithium, some anticonvulsants, thyroid hormone treatment (L-Thyroxine), select antipsychotic medications, and certain steroid hormones.

Modifiable factors for osteoporosis include:

Excessive alcohol consumption: Drinking too much alcohol leads to a higher risk for fractures. It can also cause secondary osteoporosis due to direct negative effects on bone-forming cells and nutrition.

Smoking: In addition to the harmful effects cigarettes have on the heart and lungs, smoking increases the risk of fractures and osteoporosis. Those who smoke, or have a past history of cigarette smoking, are at a higher risk of any fracture, compared to non-smokers.

Low body mass index (BMI): Lean body mass (less than 20 kg/m2) is associated with an increased risk of fracture and more bone loss.

Eating disorders: Eating disorders, such as bulimia and anorexia nervosa, often begin between adolescence and early adulthood, which is the most critical time for accumulating bone mass. These disorders can trigger the malfunction of organs and body systems, and deprive the body of nutrients needed to develop strong bones. Individuals battling eating disorders are also often at an unusually low weight and are deficient in estrogen. These factors place people with eating disorders at high risk of developing osteoporosis.

Poor nutrition: The lack of a well-balanced diet and deficiencies in important nutrients like vitamin D and calcium make individuals more prone to fractures and osteoporosis.

Not enough exercise: The absence of an exercise regimen or long-term inactivity due to bed rest or illness causes bones to weaken.

You can contact these national organizations to learn more about osteoporosis, ask specific questions, or receive additional data related to the disease:

Foundation for Osteoporosis
Research and Education (FORE)
Toll-free phone number: (888) 266-3015
Website: www.fore.org
E-mail for additional information: info@fore.org

National Institutes of Health (NIH) Osteoporosis and
Related Bone Diseases—National Resource Center
Toll-free phone number: (800) 624-BONE
Website: www.bones.nih.gov
E-mail for additional information:
NIAMSBoneInfo@mail.nih.gov

National Osteoporosis Foundation
Toll-free phone number: (800) 231-4222
Website: www.nof.org
To request additional information:
www.nof.org/request-information

Symptoms and Diagnosis of Osteoporosis

Unlike the majority of medical conditions, there are no early warning signs or glaring symptoms that point to the development of osteoporosis. In fact, the disease can be present without symptoms for several years because osteoporosis will not manifest symptoms until a bone breaks. Many people do not discover they have the disease until a painful fracture occurs. In some cases, individuals with osteoporosis may gradually start to exhibit visible signs like height loss, a protruding abdomen, or a stooped back (also called a dowager's hump) that is caused by a curvature of the spine when the vertebrae collapse.

Since osteoporosis does not have obvious symptoms, physicians may recommend doing diagnostic testing depending on the age of the person or when significant risk factors for the disease are identified.

It is possible for a routine x-ray to reveal osteoporosis because bones that are affected by the disease appear thinner and lighter in x-ray scans. Unfortunately, by the time it can be detected by an x-ray, 30% or more of the bone loss has already occurred. A standard x-ray is also not the best choice for determining bone density because the appearance of the bone can be skewed by the amount of exposure on the x-ray film. Instead, the American Medical Association, the National Osteoporosis Foundation, and other chief medical organizations recommend using a dual-energy x-ray absorptiometry scan (DXA) to properly diagnose osteoporosis. This procedure measures bone mineral density (BMD) in the spine and hip, and can be completed in less than 15 minutes. Since minerals contribute to the strength of bones, a low bone mineral density is one of the main indicators that an individual is at risk for fractures. A DXA scan is currently the only diagnostic test that is recognized as a reliable for tool for diagnosing osteoporosis.

A dual-energy x-ray absorptiometry scan compares the bone density of the patient to the average peak bone density of young adults of the same race and sex. The result, called the "T score," evaluates the bone density in terms of how many standard deviations (SD) it is below peak young adult bone mass. A bone density score of -2.5 or below confirms the presence of osteoporosis. A "T score" that is between -1 and -2.5 is indicative of osteopenia, which is bone loss that may serve as a precursor to osteoporosis, especially when combined with other risk factors.

Did You Know?

• Lifetime risks for fractures are between 40-50% in women and 13-22% in men.

• Girls obtain around 85-90% of adult bone mass by the time they are 18 years old. The same percentage is acquired in boys by the age of 20.

• Women make up 80% of the people who have osteoporosis.

• Experts predict that by 2025 osteoporosis will be responsible for almost 3 million fractures and $25.3 billion in medical costs each year.

• Any bone can be affected by osteoporosis, but the most common fractures occur in the spine, hip, and wrist.

• Osteoporosis is directly responsible for more than 1.5 million fractures in the United States every year.

• The human skeleton continues to grow from birth to the end of the teenage years, and it reaches its peak bone mass (maximum size and strength) in early adulthood.

• Statistics indicate that almost half of all women over the age of 50 will break a bone because of osteoporosis, as will one-fourth of all men over 50.

Common Treatments for Osteoporosis

The main goal of treatments for osteoporosis is to prevent bone fractures by increasing bone density and strength, and reducing bone loss. However, there are no complete cures for osteoporosis because it is difficult to rebuild bone made weak by osteoporosis. Prevention (ideally), early detection, and treatment are important to decrease the risk of osteoporotic fractures.

The following are prevention measures and treatments for osteoporosis:

• Making positive lifestyle changes like quitting smoking and drinking less alcohol reduces the modifiable risks of osteoporosis. Such changes can also strengthen the bodies of those already dealing with the disease and help lessen falls and future fractures.

• Follow a regular fitness plan that includes safe weight-bearing exercises, which are activities that make your body work against gravity. Weight-bearing exercises (such as yoga or walking), stimulate bones to retain calcium and produce more bone mass.

• Eat a more nutrient-rich (including calcium and vitamin D) and balanced diet. Reducing the amounts of animal-derived protein, salt, and caffeine in your diet is also helpful, because they all cause the body to get rid of too much calcium in the urine before the body can benefit from its bone-strengthening qualities.

• You may also choose to consult with your doctor about whether or not to take medications that stop bone loss associated with osteoporosis and increase bone strength. Some of the more common mediactions include ibandronate (Boniva), alendronate (Fosamax), risedronate (Actonel), raloxifene (Evista), calcitonin (Calcimar), zoledronate (Reclast), and denosumab (Prolia).

Vitamins and Minerals to Include in Your Diet for Bone Health

Calcium and vitamin D are the two most essential nutrients that aid in the development, health, and strength of bones. Receiving the daily requirements for them is especially important for people who have osteoporosis or are at high risk of developing the disease. Here's why:

Calcium is a mineral that is vital for building and maintaining strong, healthy bones. Your body stores close to 99% of its calcium in your bones. Children and young adults need adequate calcium intake in order to maximize the amount of calcium stored in their bones. Adults need to get the proper amount of calcium to minimize the loss of calcium stored in their bones. The National Osteoporosis Foundation (NOF) recommends a daily intake of 1,000 milligrams of calcium for children; 1,300 milligrams for teens; 1,000 milligrams for adults under 50; and 1,200 milligrams for adults over the age of 50.

Vitamin D is essential because it aids the body in properly using calcium. If your body does not get enough vitamin D or it does not absorb it well, you are at greater risk for osteoporosis and bone loss. The National Osteoporosis Foundation (NOF) recommends a daily intake of 400 IU (International Units) of vitamin D for infants; 600 IU for children teenagers, and adults under the age of 50; and 800-1,000 IU for adults 50 and older.

Some other nutrients that are beneficial to bone health are vitamins A and B12, potassium, copper, and magnesium. Below are some natural ways to get more of these important vitamins and nutrients to boost and maintain the health of your bones:

Natural Sources of Calcium:
• Milk
• Cheese
• Plain low-fat yogurt
• Sardines
• Salmon
• Any seafood that contains bones
• Turnip greens
• Spinach
• Kale
• Broccoli
• Nuts (almonds, Brazil nuts, and pecans)
• Legumes (peas, lentils, and beans)

Natural Sources of Vitamin D:
• Sunlight
• Dairy products
• Eggs
• Milk
• Tuna
• Liver oils
• Mackerel
• Cod
• Sea bass

Natural Sources of Vitamin A:
• Dairy products
• Milk
• Eggs
• Yellow vegetables (summer squash)
• Carrots
• Liver
• Green leafy vegetables (kale, spinach, greens, and romaine lettuce)
• Fruits (cantaloupe, tomatoes, and apricots)

Natural Sources of Vitamin B12:
• Liver
• Lean beef
• Clams
• Salmon
• Haddock
• Trout
• Cheese
• Dairy
• Eggs

Natural Sources of Potassium:
• Milk
• Green leafy vegetables (romaine lettuce, spinach, Swiss chard, and greens)
• Broccoli
• Lentils
• Winter squash
• Fruits (tomatoes, cantaloupe, avocado, oranges, and strawberries)
• Snapper
• Halibut
• Scallops
• Soy
• Potatoes (white and sweet varieties)

Natural Sources of Copper:
• Vegetables
• Liver
• Legumes
• Nuts
• Seeds
• Beans

Natural Sources of Magnesium:
- Brazil nuts
- Seeds (sunflower seeds, pumpkin seeds, and sesame seeds)
- Bananas
- Legumes
- Tofu
- Green leafy vegetables (spinach, Swiss chard, and kelp)
- Whole grains (barley, brown rice, and oats)

CHAPTER 2

THE BENEFITS OF YOGA

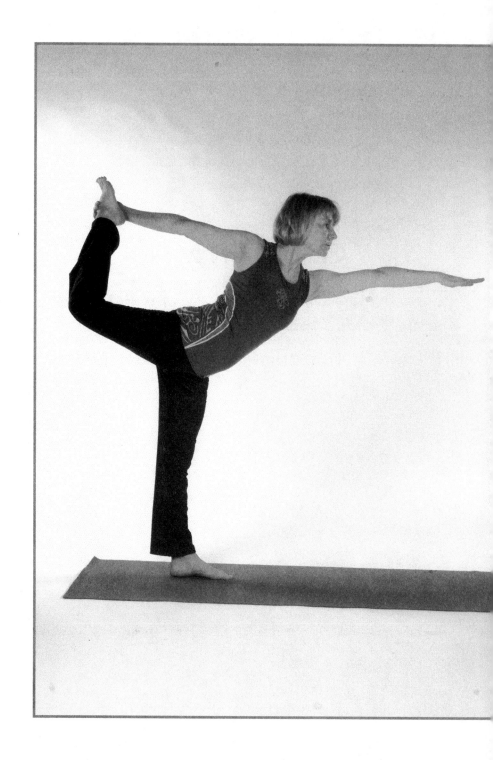

Bone is living tissue, so it responds to exercise by growing stronger, in much the same way muscles do. While exercise cannot replace bone that has already been lost, it does make bones denser and stronger when you make them work. The two types of exercises that work best for building and maintaining bone density are weight-bearing and muscle-strengthening exercises.

Weight-bearing exercises, ones that apply pressure on bones, help stimulate the bones to hold on to calcium and create more bone mass. Common examples are walking, jogging, or stair climbing. However, not all weight-bearing exercises have to be high-impact. If you have osteoporosis or are at high risk of developing the disease, it is essential to choose exercises that are safe for you and gentler on your bones.

Muscle-strengthening exercises include activities that use your body, weights, or some other type of resistance against gravity. Examples of exercises that strengthen muscles are lifting weights and using resistance bands. The spine needs the support of the muscles and tendons that surround it. Keeping those muscles and tendons flexible and strong helps the spine to remain upright and protects it from many injuries. These exercises also help with prevention and management of osteoporosis because bones are strengthened by the force the nearby muscles put on them. Therefore, the stronger the muscles become, the more your bones are strengthened by them.

Yoga combines both weight-bearing exercises and muscle-strengthening exercises, making it a wise choice for people with osteoporosis. It also enhances bone-building for both the upper and lower body, instead of focusing on one or the other like many forms of exercise do. Plus, yoga is low-impact so there is less danger of stress fractures or falls that often accompany more high-impact forms of exercise.

The practice also offers many other benefits, such as relieving pain, stress, and anxiety. It also improves strength, flexibility, posture, balance, and coordination:

Offers relief from pain, stress and anxiety: Yoga is effective in alleviating pain, and reducing stress and anxiety, which can compromise systems in your body and affect functions like immunity and digestion. Yoga practices such as meditation help the individual focus on something other than what he or she feels. It also allows the entire body to relax and get the rest it needs to replenish itself.

Strengthens muscles and increases flexibility: Strong and flexible muscles boost the strength of the bones they surround and offer them added protection. While muscles should be strong, ones that are too large (like ones acquired from heavy weightlifting) may cause too much strain on the brittle bones of someone with osteoporosis. Yoga provides a way to strengthen muscles and build flexibility without making them too bulky. Strengthening your muscles, particularly those in the back and shoulders, also helps improve your posture.

Promotes good posture: Good posture is important for maintaining a strong, healthy, and flexible spine. Yoga exercises, especially the seated and standing poses, help focus on posture and the alignment of the spine. Proper posture relieves some of the pressure off the spine and reduces the back pain often associated with osteoporosis. Practicing good posture can also keep kyphosis (the curve of the upper back caused by broken bones in the spine) to a minimum.

Creates balance and coordination: It is beneficial for individuals who have osteoporosis to improve balance and coordination. Injuries incurred from falling present a huge risk for people with osteoporosis. Yoga helps increase your balance and coordination, which will make you more stable on your feet and reduce the number of falls you take.

Yoga and the Mind-Body Connection

Yoga is a mind-body kind of exercise that helps you stay fit and relaxed, and is also beneficial for managing chronic pain associated with illnesses like osteoporosis. Since yoga combines movement and conscious breathing exercises, it helps you focus both on what your body is physically doing and what is occurring internally. As the root "yuj" (meaning unity or yoke) implies, yoga is an exercise form that seeks to unify the mind and body. When that union takes place, it brings with it a wealth of therapeutic benefits.

The practice of yoga can be traced back to over 5000 years ago, to a time when monks in India (called yogi) secluded themselves and sat for hours in deep meditation in an attempt to create strong, disease-free bodies. While they found the meditation good for the mind, their sore bodies would not allow them to stay in the same position for extended periods. Instead, they had to change positions while still focusing on their meditation. Over time, more structured yoga postures stemmed from these early practices and addressed specific needs in the body as well as the mind.

Today, yoga is used in many therapeutic ways, such as to detoxify, relieve anxiety and depression, realign musculature, strengthen muscles, create flexibility, and manage chronic pain.

"Yoga teaches us to cure what need not be endured, and endure what cannot be cured."
—B.K.S. Iyengar

Read more about yoga and its benefits on these sites:

American Yoga Association
www.americanyogaassociation.org

International Association of Yoga Therapists
www.iayt.org

Meditation Tips for Beginners

Yoga offers meditation and controlled breathing techniques that can be used effectively to manage the pain associated with your osteoporosis and refocus your thoughts. Meditating for only a few minutes each day can help.

Here are a few quick tips for meditation beginners:

• Take the time to stretch out first. Loosening muscles and tendons before beginning allows you to sit or lie down more comfortably.

• Make it a formal practice by setting aside a specific time and place to devote to your meditation.

•Focus on your breathing. Slowing your breathing helps your mind and body to relax and prepare for meditation.

• Meditate in the morning. It is usually quieter in the morning, and your mind has not yet had the chance to get cluttered. It will also help work out any kinks in your body from sleeping. And it's always great to start your day with focus!

• Find a time and place to meditate where you will not be disturbed.

• Enlist the help of instructional videos or calming music if they help you relax more.

• Light a candle and use it as a focal point, instead of closing your eyes. Focusing on the light causes you to strengthen your attention.

• Be aware of your body and how it feels in both its normal and relaxed states, and embrace the differences.

• Experiment with different types of meditation and different positions. You won't know which methods work best for you until you try them.

• Have a purpose behind your meditation, such as pain management or feeling more focused on a specific issue you must deal with.

• Push aside any feelings of doubt, frustration, and stress about whether or not you are doing it right. It is counterproductive to your meditation.

• Relax and relish in your mind's incredible ability to focus and care for your body through meditation.

• Remember your meditation and breathing techniques throughout the day. A few well-placed cleansing breaths will do wonders for your mind and body.

Some of the most commonly recommended yoga poses for osteoporosis can be found in this book, including:

Cobra
Corpse
Downward-Facing Dog
Ear to Shoulder
Mountain
Neck Rolls
Reverse Warrior
Tree
Upward-Facing Dog
Warrior I
Warrior II
Warrior III

CHAPTER 3

SAFETY PRECAUTIONS

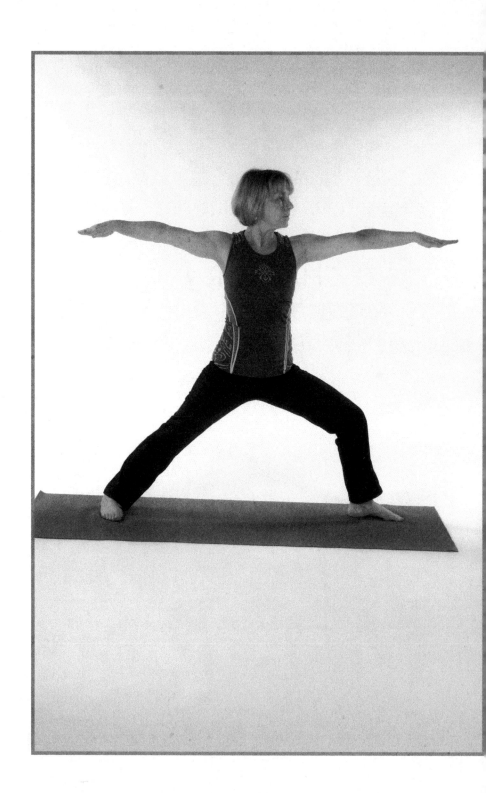

L earning the proper ways to move, sit, and stand can help you stay mobile and active, while protecting against future fractures. Maintaining good posture helps combat against curvature of the spine that is sometimes associated with osteoporosis and spinal fractures. Alignment (which is the way the head, shoulders, spine, hips, knees, and ankles line up with each other) is important for sustaining proper posture. When the body is properly aligned, it also puts less stress on the spine and results in fewer bone breaks.

To keep proper alignment, the following positions or movements should be avoided as much as possible:

• Bending forward from the waist

• Twisting the spine to the point of strain

• Slumping over with your head forward

• Twisting the trunk and bending forward when vacuuming, lifting, coughing, or sneezing

• Reaching too far (such as straining to reach for something on a high shelf)

Even though an active lifestyle is healthy, there are some exercises that may actually cause more harm than good. If you have osteoporosis or any past broken bones in the spine, it is best to avoid exercises that involve bending over from the waist (like toe-touches, abdominal crunches, and sit-ups). When you bow forward at the waist, the shoulders and back become rounded and can increase the risk of fracturing the spine. Some forms of exercise that involve bending and twisting motions can be modified to gain the benefits from them, while not placing too much stress on the spine and increasing the likelihood of fractures. Yoga is one beneficial practice that can be safely modified to aid people who have osteoporosis. It's important to remember that as your body changes and matures, the way you practice yoga must also change. Approach your yoga exercises with gentleness and acceptance of the body you have now, and allow it to work safely for you.

Follow these guidelines to ensure safety when practicing yoga exercises for osteoporosis:

• It is always recommended that you talk to your doctor before starting an exercise program. This is especially true if you know you have osteoporosis or bone loss.

• Once you have the approval of your doctor, start the exercise program and ease into the more difficult moves. These gentle yoga exercises are intended to strengthen your body and relieve some of the symptoms associated with your osteoporosis, not aggravate them.

• If you are new to yoga, you may find it best to start by holding the poses for only a few long, deep breaths. As you progress and feel more comfortable, you can begin to hold the poses for longer.

• If you already have osteoporosis, use extreme caution when doing exercises that involve bending and twisting at the waist. These types of motions can put you at risk of fracture. Talk to a doctor, physical therapist, or trainer about possible modified versions.

• Concentrate more on maintaining proper alignment while doing your yoga exercises, and focus less on pushing over your limits. Recognize your limitations and respect them. Trying to surpass your limits may inflict unnecessary pain or risk of injury.

• Since everyone has varying degrees of bone loss, flexibility, and pain associated with osteoporosis and previous fractures, it is important not to gauge your level of difficulty against someone else's. Practice the yoga exercises to the degree that you can perform them comfortably and safely for your own body.

• If any of the yoga moves cause you pain in your bones or joints, listen to your body and stop immediately.

Yoga Postures to Avoid When Dealing with Osteoporosis or Bone Loss

• Do not flex the spine forward to stretch abdominal muscles, back, or legs. There are recycling poses that will accomplish similar goals without risking injury.

• Exercise extreme caution when approaching backbends, and avoid overarching your back. If you can safely do so, try backbends that are gently supported.

• Never support your whole body weight with just your hands. Wrist fractures are very common with osteoporosis. Instead, consider other safer yoga movements that help build the muscles and bones in your wrists and arms.

• Avoid inversions, poses that involve you supporting yourself while being upside down. Restorative poses allow you to enjoy some of the same benefits without inverting yourself.

• Do not twist the spine in any way that uses leverage for rotation. Introduce poses that involve rotations into your exercise routine slowly and use gentle movements without force.

•Avoid doing standing poses and balances without the support of a person, wall, or chair close by. These poses work great but also increase the risk of fracture due to balance issues.

How to Protect Against Injuries
Associated with Falling

Since individuals with osteoporosis or bone loss need to avoid unnecessary injuries, below is a list of helpful reminders on how to protect from falls and reduce the risks of future fractures.

When you are outdoors:
• Use a cane, walker, or arm of a loved one to lend support.
• Wear shoes with rubber soles and good traction to prevent slipping.
• Carry a shoulder bag or fanny pack to keep your hands free.
• Sprinkle salt or kitty litter on icy walkways in the winter months.
• Try to walk in the grass or around icy or wet sidewalks.

When you are indoors:
• Keep rooms well-lit. You may also consider installing night-lights in halls, stairways, and dimly lit areas.
• Use a rubber bath mat in the shower or bathtub to protect against slipping.
• Install grab bars in the bathroom near the toilet, tub, and shower.
• Do not walk in slippers, stockings, or socks in the house. Instead, wear low-heeled shoes that offer more support and less slipping.
• Lay carpet runners on slippery floors. Be sure to tack them down or attach them with skid-proof backing.
• Make sure stairwells are lit and have railings on both sides. Don't forget to use them!
• Keep clutter to a minimum to avoid tripping hazards, especially on the floors and high-traffic areas.
• Store a flashlight by your bed in case you need to get up in the night.
• Buy a cordless phone and always keep it nearby. You won't have to rush to answer it, and it will be handy if you do fall and need to call for assistance.

CHAPTER 4

THE POSES

MOUNTAIN

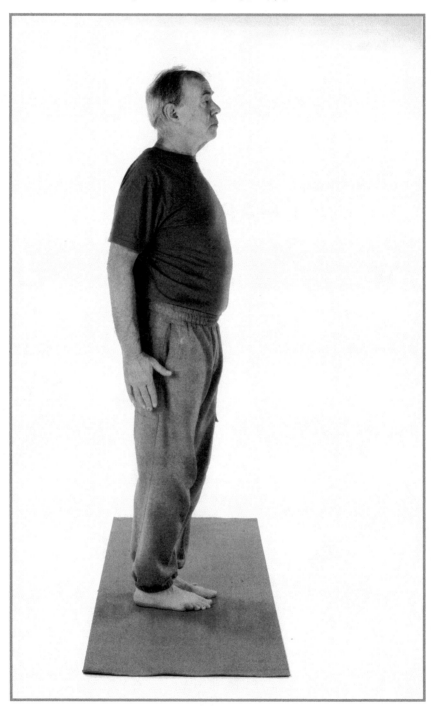

MODIFICATION

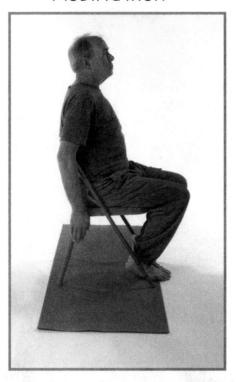

Stand with your big toes touching. Roll your shoulders up, back, and down—this movement places your shoulder blades on your back. Try to find your balance over the arches of your feet by rocking back and forth from the balls of your feet to the heels. Then build your body up from your feet and through your calves, pulling your kneecaps up, tightening your thighs, and tucking your tailbone under. Your chin should be centered with your chest. Exhale and pull up on your pelvic floor. On the next exhale, pull your stomach up and back (this will create strength in your abdominals). This "lock" in the abdominals should be used in all standing postures.

For the chair variation, sit upright in a chair with your legs and feet together and your arms at your sides. Roll your shoulders up, back, and down, then follow the directions to create a "lock" in your abdominals.

REVERSE WARRIOR

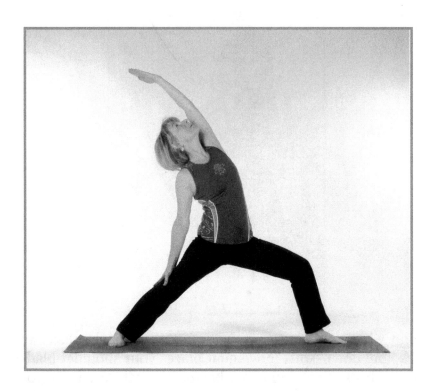

Start in Warrior II pose, facing to the right (your legs will not move throughout this sequence). Position your arms out in a 'T' position. On the inhale, drop your left hand down to your left leg as you raise your right arm straight up. Exhale and bend your right arm over your head as you bend your torso back, stretching the right side of your body up and back. Hold for five breaths. Repeat on the left side.

MODIFICATION

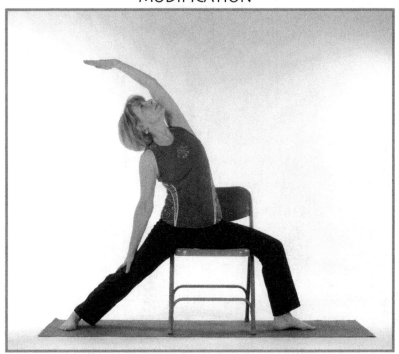

For the chair variation, start by sitting on a chair. Straddle the chair, bending your right knee as you turn your right foot out 90 degrees. Extend your left leg out straight and then follow the arm directions.

WARM-UP FORWARD BEND

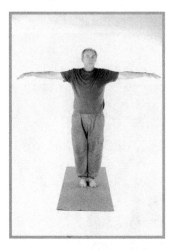

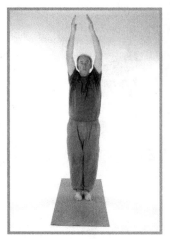

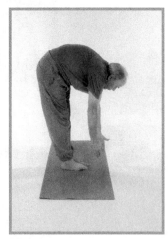

Stand with your feet together in Mountain pose. On the in-hale, sweep your arms up and over your head. Reach up and then back, stretching through both sides of your torso with your weight in your heels. On the exhale, swan-dive down into a forward bend with your arms out to your sides, leading with your chin and chest. Sweep your hands close to the floor and inhale all the way up and back again. Repeat five to six times.

MODIFICATION

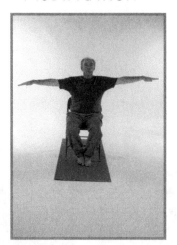

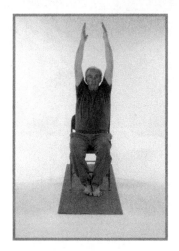
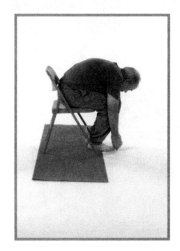

For the chair variation, sit in the chair and face forward with your legs and feet together. Sweep your arms up and then on the exhale, bend down over your legs. On the inhale, come up and reach back. In the beginning, your back may be rounded. As you gain strength, try to come down and up with a straight back.

Note: This pose should be done from the hips, not the waist. As always, use caution and be sure to "listen" to your body—if the pose becomes too difficult, stop or switch to a more gentle variation.

NECK ROLLS

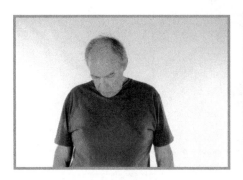
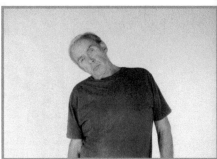

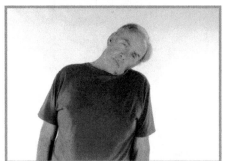
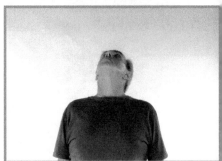

Stand with your feet together in Mountain pose, keeping your shoulders relaxed. Roll your neck to the right, circling slowly all the way around. Go four or five times one way, then reverse and circle another four or five times in the other direction.

Images are shown clockwise.

EAR TO SHOULDER

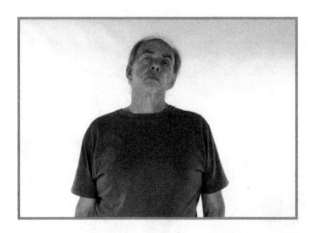

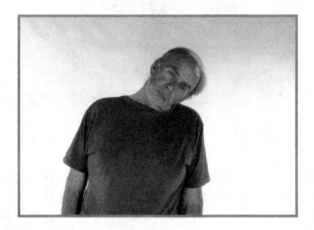

Stand with your feet together in Mountain pose. Drop your left ear to your left shoulder and then bring your right ear to your right shoulder.

HALF MOON

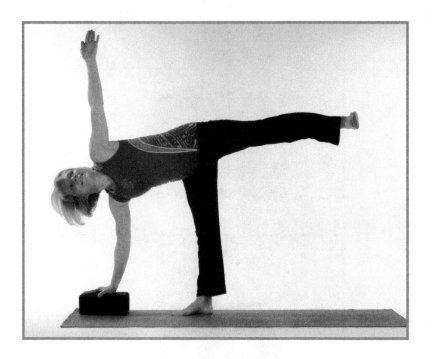

Beginners should use a block for this pose, placing the block by your right foot. Begin with your feet together in Mountain pose in the middle of the mat. Take a wide-legged stance, turn your right foot out 90 degrees, and bend your right knee so that your chest is resting on your right thigh. Place the block in your hand and bring it at least six inches in front of your right foot, keeping it in line with your baby toe. On the inhale, straighten your right leg while lifting your left. Keep your weight in your right leg and hand. Tighten your abdominals and both legs (the block has three levels, so start at the highest level and as you gain strength and balance use the lower levels).

MODIFICATION

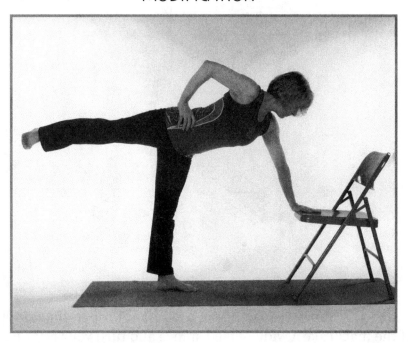

Place your left hand on your waist and work up to five full breaths. As this pose becomes easier, you may wish to increase the intensity by raising your left arm up towards the ceiling while turning your head to look up at your hand. You may also use a different height on the block, working towards the goal of placing your hand on the floor. Repeat on the left side.

For the chair variation, place a chair six to ten inches away from your right foot. In a wide-legged stance, proceed as described above, placing your hand on the chair for balance.

LATERAL STRETCH

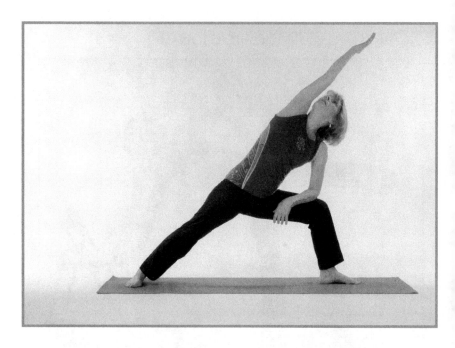

Start with your feet together in Mountain pose in the middle of the mat. Take a wide-legged stance and turn your right foot out 90 degrees. On the exhale, bend your right knee, keeping the outside of your left foot on the floor. On the next exhale, drop your right forearm to your thigh and, on the inhale, raise your left arm up. On the next exhale, stretch your left arm over your head while stretching from your left foot through your leg, hips, ribs and out from the fingertips of your left hand. With your palm facing down, turn your head to look at your palm—this keeps your neck in line with your spine. Hold for five breaths and repeat on the left side. As you gain strength in your legs, you may try this by using a block on the outside of your right foot. On the exhale, place your right hand down to the block and proceed as before. This pose may also be done with a chair by straddling the chair, positioning your legs in Warrior II (see page 44) and then proceeding with the arm movements.

HANDS UNDER TOES

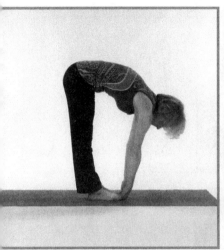
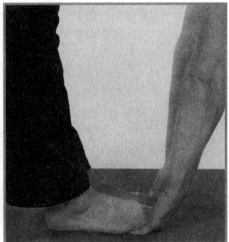

Start with your feet together in Mountain pose. On the inhale, sweep your arms widely up and back. On the exhale, swandive down and bring your fingers under your toes, bending your knees as much as needed. On the inhale, raise your head and chest, keeping your fingers in place. On the exhale, lower your head. Repeat four to five times.

Note: This pose should be done from the hips, not the waist. As always, use caution and be sure to "listen" to your body—if the pose becomes too difficult, stop or switch to a more gentle variation.

WARRIOR 1

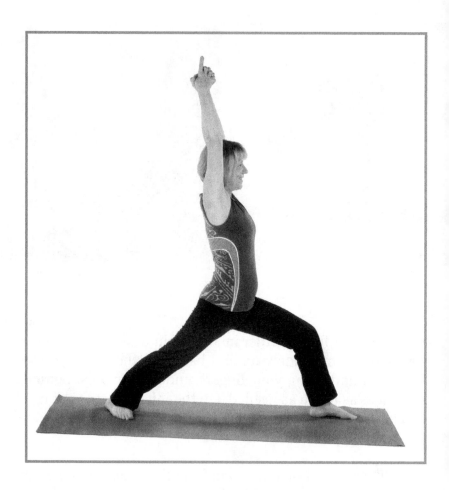

Start with your feet together in Mountain pose. Take a wide-legged stance and turn your right foot out 90 degrees. Turn to face over your right foot with your shoulders and your hips. On the exhale, bend your right knee. On the inhale, raise your arms over your head and interlock your fingers. For increased intensity (not pictured), look up at your hands and hold for five breaths. Repeat on the left side.

MODIFICATION

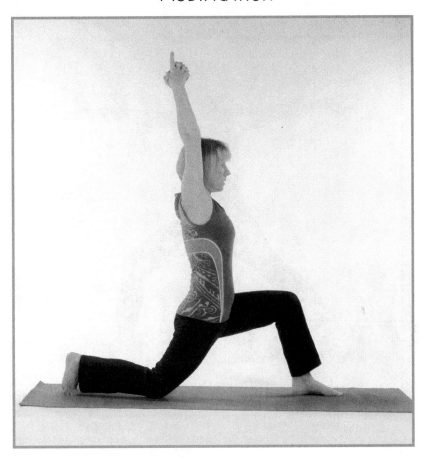

If this seems difficult, you may drop your back knee to the floor until you gain balance and strength.

WARRIOR II

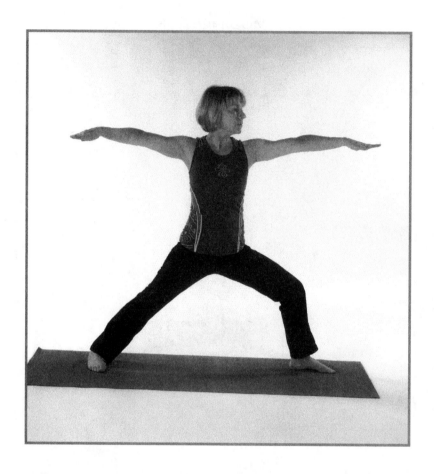

Start with your feet together in Mountain pose. Take a wide-legged stance and, on the exhale, turn your right foot out 90 degrees, keeping your hips and shoulders facing forward. On the inhale, raise your arms into a 'T' position. On the next exhale, bend your right knee over your ankle. Your weight should be on the outside of your left foot as you pull up in your inner left thigh. Your focal point will be at the fingertips of your right hand. Hold for five breaths. Repeat on the left side.

MODIFICATION

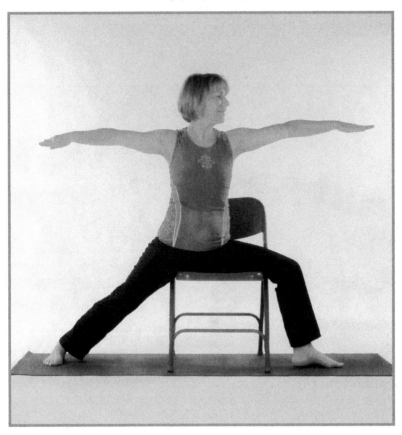

For the chair variation, sit on a chair and come to a straddle
position. Bend your right knee and turn your right foot out 90
degrees. Extend your left leg out straight. On the inhale, raise
your arms up and hold for five breaths.

WARRIOR III

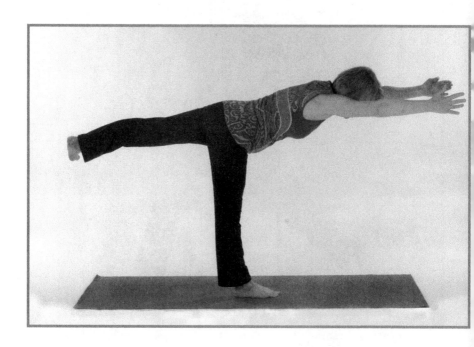

Start with your feet together, placing your weight on your left foot. On the inhale, raise your arms shoulder-width over your head. On the exhale, come forward with your torso and raise your right leg behind, keeping your hips parallel. Tighten your left leg and your abdominal muscles to hold your body up. Work up to five breaths. Repeat on the left side.

MODIFICATION

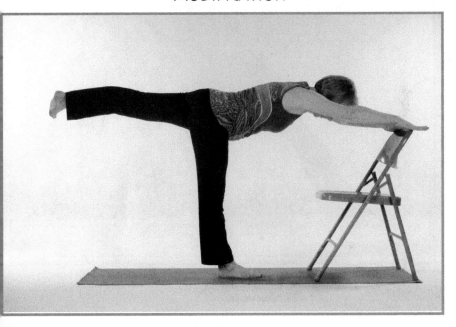

If this seems difficult, the pose can also be performed with your hands against the wall or on a chair, as shown.

DOWNWARD-FACING DOG

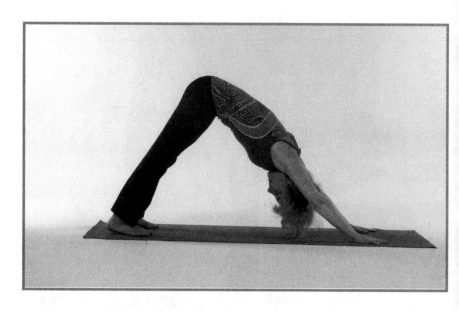

Start with your feet together in Mountain pose. On the inhale, raise your arms wide, up and back. On the exhale, come forward and bring your face to your knees, bending your knees as much as needed to bring your palms to the floor. On the exhale, raise your right leg and place it behind you into a runner's pose. Raise your left leg and take it back to meet the right (your feet can be together or hip-width apart). Push back through your hands and arms until you are in an inverted 'V' position. Your head should be between your arms, with your hips pushing up and heels pushing down. Your weight will be in your feet, palms, and index fingers. Hold for five breaths. To come up, step forward.

MODIFICATION

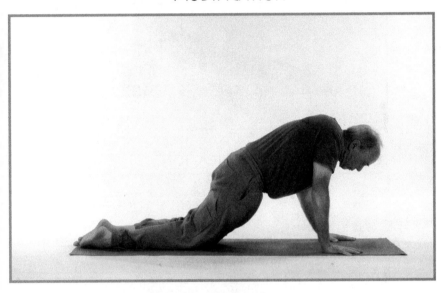

This may also be done by starting in a kneeling position on your hands and knees (in a tabletop position), then curling your toes under and pushing back into an inverted 'V' position.

UPWARD-FACING DOG

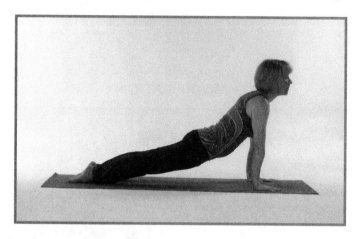

MODIFICATION

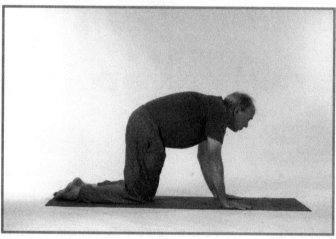

Start by lying on the mat on your stomach, with your forehead on the floor. Bring your hands under your shoulders, keeping your elbows close to your body and your legs and feet together. On the inhale, push up with your arms, raise your head, then roll your shoulders up and back, while pushing against your hands. Rising up, lift your hips and thighs off the mat so that your weight is on the top of your feet and in your hands. If this is difficult, you can raise up to your knees, working up to rising to your feet. Work up to five breaths.

FULL SQUAT

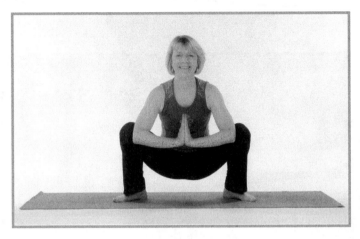

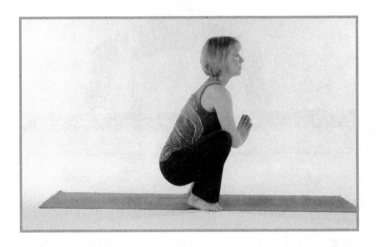

Start with your feet a little more than hip-width apart and your toes pointing out (your feet can be out as far as the edge of the mat). Bring your hands together in prayer position and bend your knees, coming down as far as you can while keeping the soles of your feet on the ground. Work up to five breaths. To come up, place your hands on the floor and straighten your legs, then slowly roll your spine up.

YOGA SQUAT/FORWARD BEND

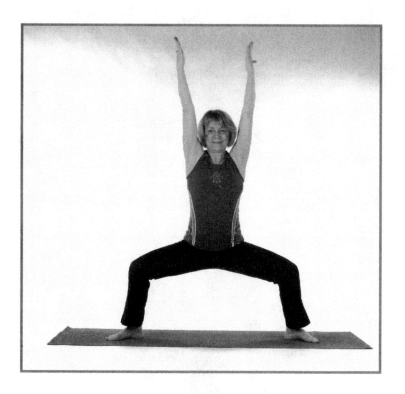

Stand in a wide-legged stance with your feet pointing out. On the inhale, bend your knees and come down halfway while raising your arms into a wide 'V' position.

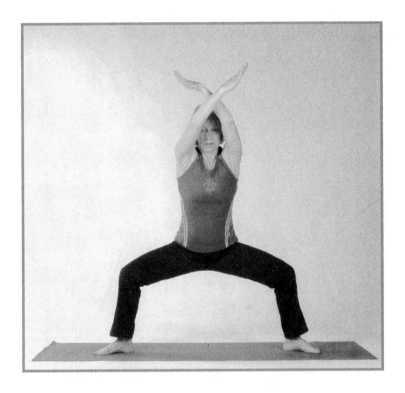

On the exhale, keep your legs where they are and cross your arms above your head.

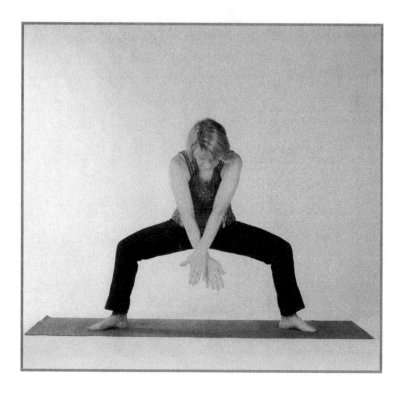

Bend forward halfway, with your arms crossed in front of your body.

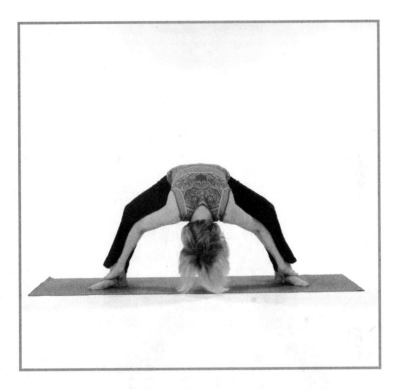

Continue to bend forward and bring your hands to your ankles and your elbows to your knees.

On the next inhale, rise back up into the "V" position. On the exhale, lower down again. Repeat four to five times.

Note: This pose should be done from the hips, not the waist. Once your hands are under your toes, raise your head to keep your spine in alignment and prevent a "hump" in your back.

This pose can also be done with your hands on a chair so that you can straighten your back. As always, use caution and be sure to "listen" to the body—if the pose becomes too difficult, stop or switch to a more gentle variation.

TRIANGLE

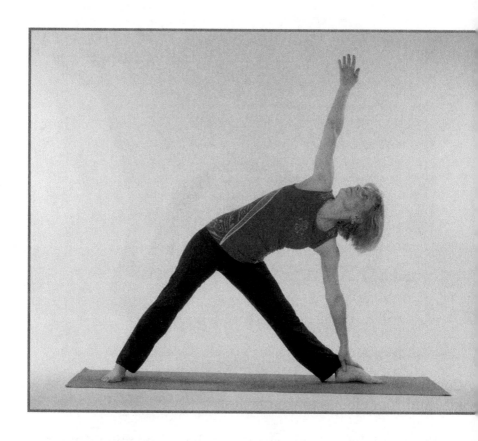

Start with your feet together in Mountain pose in the middle of the mat. Take a wide-legged stance and turn your right foot out 90 degrees. On the inhale, raise your arms into a 'T' position, extending them out from your shoulders. On the exhale, reach your right arm up, out, and down while pulling in on your right hip (this is a lunge movement to the right). Bring your right hand to rest on your leg wherever it goes easily (this means your hand may be as high as your knee since you are aiming for alignment of your shoulder over your leg).

MODIFICATION

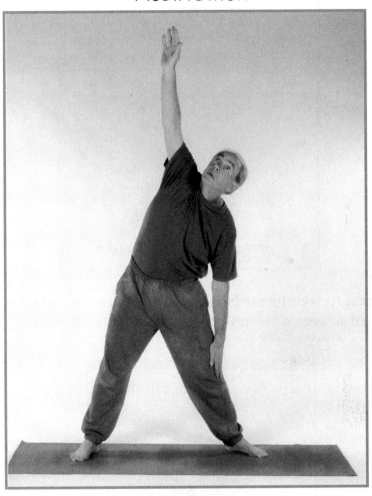

On the next breath, reach your left arm up towards the ceiling, keeping both legs straight (a block may be used here by placing it on the outside of your right foot and extending out and then down to the block). Try to turn your head to look up at your left hand, this will keep you neck in line with the spine. Hold for five breaths.

REVERSE TRIANGLE

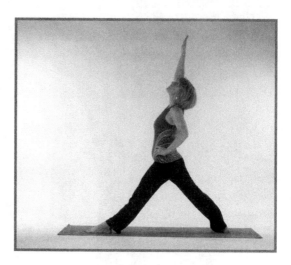

Start with your feet together in Mountain pose. Take a wide-legged stance and turn your right foot out 90 degrees.

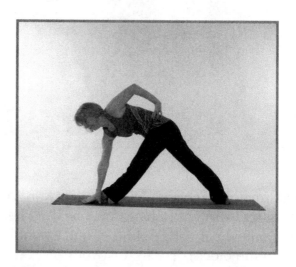

Place the block (if using) on the outside of your right foot and then turn your body to face over your right foot with both hips and shoulders facing right. Place your right hand on your hip.

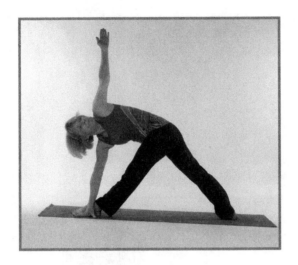

On the inhale, raise your left arm up and back, stretching back. On the exhale, start the twist as you come forward, placing your left hand to your knee, the block, or the floor. Hold for five breaths. For increased intensity, raise your right arm towards the ceiling while looking up at your hand.

When using the block, remember that it has three heights and beginners should start with the highest level.

Note: This pose should be done from the hips, not the waist. As always, use caution and be sure to "listen" to the body—if the pose becomes too difficult, stop or switch to a more gentle variation.

TREE

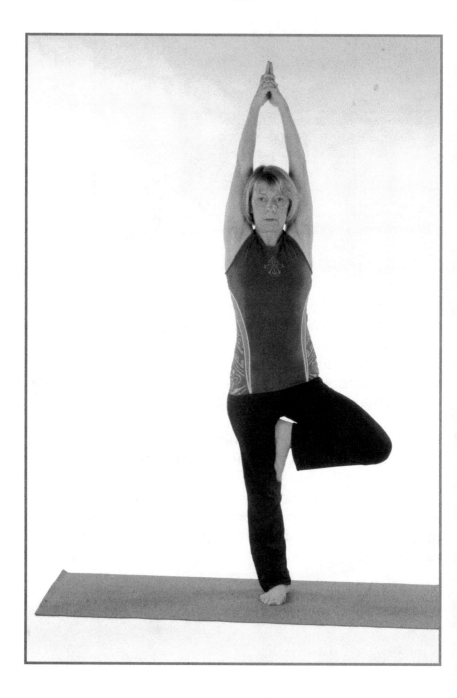

MODIFICATION 1

MODIFICATION 2

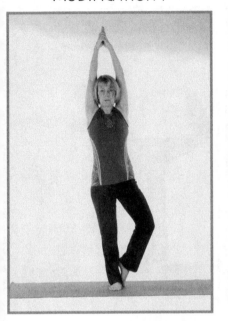

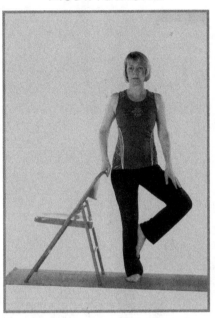

Start with your feet together in Mountain pose. Shift your weight to your right leg and raise your left leg, placing the sole of your left foot on the inside of your right leg. Try to place your left foot as high as possible on your right leg, taking care not to place it on the inside of your knee (you may use a chair, as shown, or the wall to hold on to in the beginning). Bring your hands together in the center of your chest, with your hands in prayer position. Hold for five breaths. For increased intensity, raise your arms overhead, keeping your hands together and bringing your arms as close to your ears as possible.

DANCING SHIVA

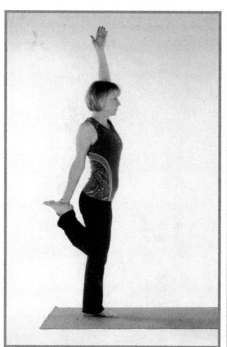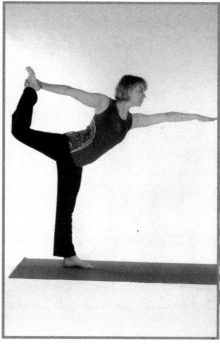

Start with your feet together in Mountain pose. Shift your weight to your right leg and raise your left leg, bending at the knee. Bring your left foot up behind you and grab your foot with your palm facing up in the inside of your foot. You may hold here or, for increased intensity, raise your right arm straight up and on the exhale, bring your arm forward then extend your left leg back and up. Work up to five breaths. Repeat on the left side.

MODIFICATION

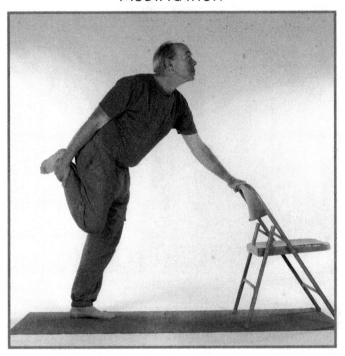

For the chair variation, place a chair arms-length in front of your body and proceed as described, placing your hand on the back of the chair for balance.

STANDING LEG LIFT

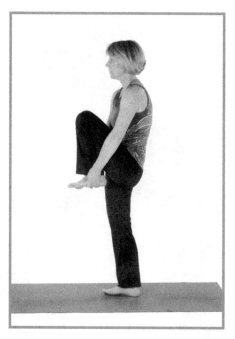

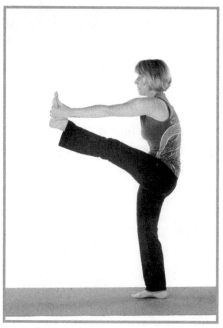

MODIFICATION 1

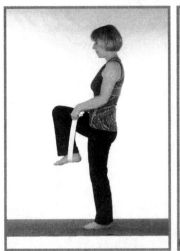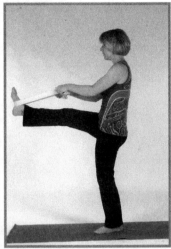

MODIFICATION 2

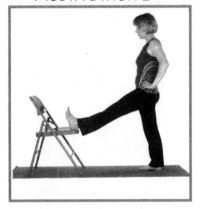

Start with your feet together in Mountain pose, placing your weight on your left leg. Bend your right knee and wrap a strap under your right foot. Hold the strap in your right hand and straighten your right leg out in front of your body. For increased intensity (not pictured), bring your right leg out to the right and use your left arm for balance by placing it out to the left. Work up to five or six breaths. Repeat on the other side. This may also be done using a chair by placing your foot on the chair. As you gain balance and strength, move the strap as described. Once this becomes easy to perform with the strap, try bending your knee and grabbing your foot in your hands, then extend out.

COBRA

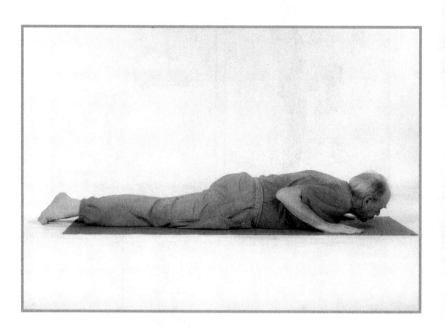

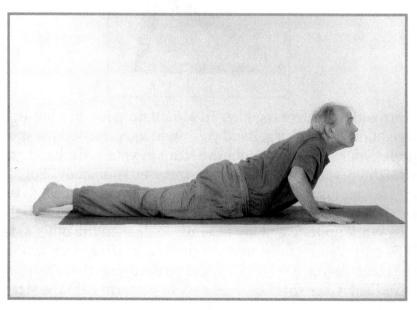

MODIFICATION

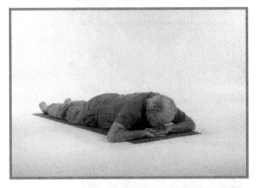

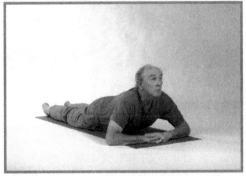

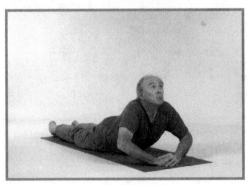

Start by lying on the mat on your stomach. Bring your feet and legs together and keep your forehead to the floor. Bring your hands under your shoulders and on the inhale, push your body up with your arms and roll your shoulders up and back while expanding your chest and keeping your hips on the floor (this will work the lower back). Hold for three full breaths and release down. Come up again and hold for three more full breaths.

HERO

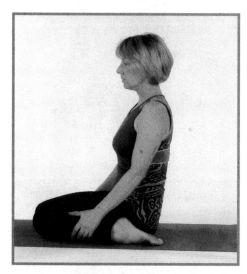

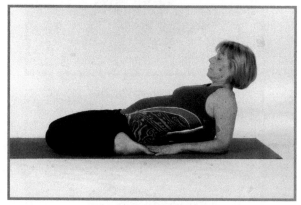

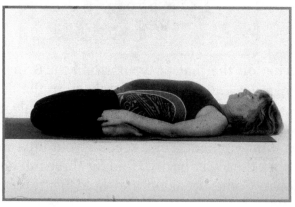

MODIFICATION

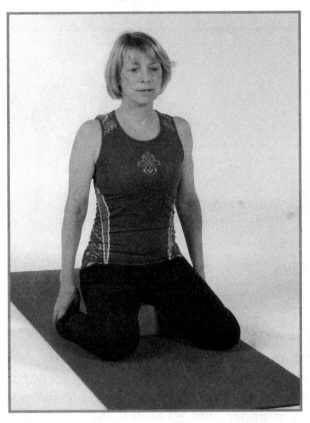

Come onto your knees. Try to sit back between your legs. If this is difficult, use a blanket under your knees or rest your sitting bone on a block (start by using the highest level and lower as you become more flexible), opening up in your ankles, knees, and hips. For increased intensity, you can bring your sitting bone to the floor and try to lean back onto your elbows, eventually resting your torso on the floor.

PLANK

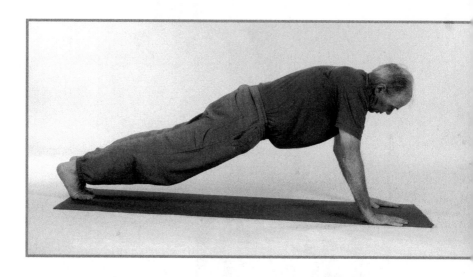

Start with your feet together in Mountain pose. On the inhale, sweep your arms up. On the exhale, bend forward and swan-dive down. Bend your knees as needed to place your hands on the floor under your shoulders. Step your feet back and create a straight line with your body. Hold for five breaths. For increased intensity (not pictured), you may perform a side plank. Make sure your right hand is directly under your right shoulder and roll over onto the right side, trying to stack your feet one on top of the other. You can then also try to raise your left arm or keep it at your waist. Come back to the center plank and roll onto the left side (if performing the side plank).

MODIFICATION

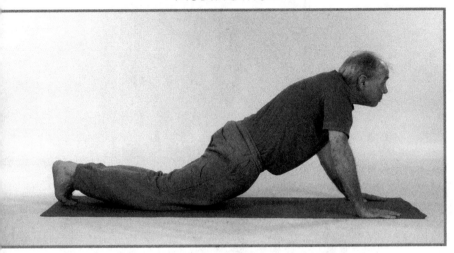

For beginners, start on your hands and knees (in a tabletop position) and step one foot back at a time until you can hold the pose with both feet back.

CHILD

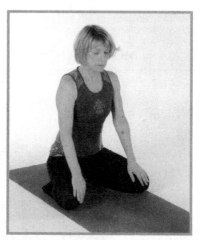

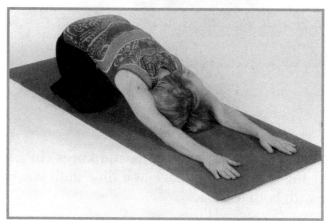

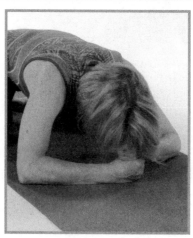

MODIFICATION 1

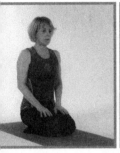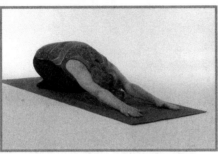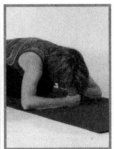

MODIFICATION 2

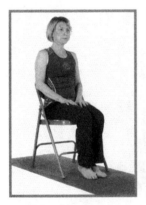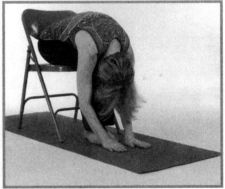

Kneel on the mat, separate your knees, and sit back on your heels (you may also keep your knees together if this is uncomfortable). Bring your body forward, trying to touch your forehead to the floor (if this is difficult, make a fist with your hands and place your forehead on your fists).

For the chair variation, sit with your legs and feet together and roll forward with your arms by your legs and your hands at your feet.

CAT AND DOG

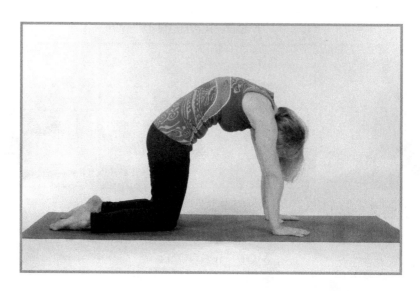

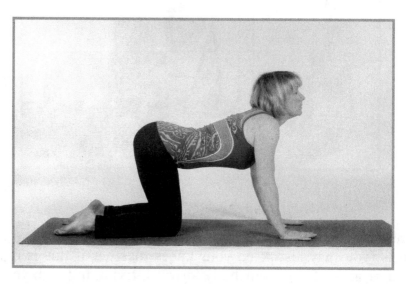

Start on all fours with your hands under your shoulders and your knees under your hips. On the exhale, round your back up to arch like a cat and bring your hips forward. Bring your chin to your chest. On the inhale, drop your belly and raise your head, pushing your sitting bones back and up. Repeat four to five times with your breath.

CORPSE

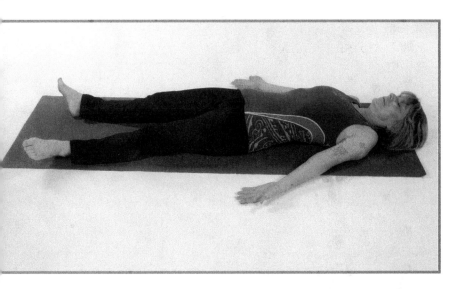

Lie on your back, with your arms extended out from your body and your palms facing up. Keep your legs a little more than hip-width apart to remove any tension from your hips. Close your eyes, bring your chin into the center of your chest, and keep your shoulders relaxed and away from your ears. Breathe deeply into your belly, letting your belly rise and fall with each breath. This pose is recommended at the end of your session to give your body a chance to relax and to allow the previous work from the poses to settle.

CHAPTER 5

GENTLE FLOWS FOR OSTEOPOROSIS

BALANCE

POSE	PAGE	EQUIPMENT
Mountain	30	chair (optional)
Standing Leg Lift	64	chair or strap (optional)
Dancing Shiva	62	chair (optional)
Tree	60	chair (optional)
Warrior III	46	chair (optional)
Corpse	75	

LEG STRENGTH

POSE	PAGE	EQUIPMENT
Mountain	30	chair (optional)
Warrior I	42	
Warrior II	44	chair (optional)
Reverse Warrior	32	chair (optional)
Lateral Stretch	40	block (optional)
Yoga Squat/Forward Bend	52	chair (optional)
Corpse	75	

UPPER BODY STRENGTH

POSE	PAGE	EQUIPMENT
Mountain	30	chair (optional)
Downward-Facing Dog	48	
Plank	70	
Cobra	66	
Upward-Facing Dog	50	
Corpse	75	

SPINE FLEXIBILITY

POSE	PAGE	EQUIPMENT
Mountain	30	chair (optional)
Warrior II	44	chair (optional)
Reverse Warrior	32	chair (optional)
Triangle	56	block (optional)
Reverse Triangle	58	block (optional)
Cat and Dog	74	
Corpse	75	

HIP STRENGTH & FLEXIBILITY

POSE	PAGE	EQUIPMENT
Mountain	30	chair (optional)
Yoga Squat/Forward Bend	52	chair (optional)
Full Squat	51	
Tree	60	chair (optional)
Lateral Stretch	40	block (optional)
Corpse	75	

REFERENCES

American Yoga Association
www.americanyogaassociation.org

Foundation for Osteoporosis Research
and Education (FORE)
www.fore.org

International Osteoporosis Foundation
www.iofbonehealth.org

National Institute of Aging
www.nia.nih.gov

National Institutes of Health: Osteoporosis and
Related Bone Diseases—National Resource Center
www.bones.nih.gov

National Osteoporosis Foundation
www.nof.org

Women's Health
www.womenshealth.gov

World's Healthiest Foods
whfoods.org

Yoga Journal
www.yogajournal.com

LAURIE SANFORD

Laurie Sanford has practiced yoga for 14 years and is certified under Rob Greenberg, owner of the Yoga for Peace Studio in Margaretville, NY. She has been teaching for eight years and currently provides yoga instruction to adults. Laurie has trained at the Kripalu Center for Yoga and Health, as well as the Himalayan Institute. She currently resides with her husband and daughter in the Catskill Mountains, where they run a weekly newspaper.

JO BRIELYN

Jo Brielyn is a freelance writer and author. She is a contributing writer for Hatherleigh Press and has published works in several print and online publications. Jo also owns and maintains the Creative Kids Ideas (www.creativekidsideas.com) and Good for Your Health (www.good-for-your-health.com) websites. For more information about Jo's upcoming projects or to contact her, visit www.JoBrielyn.com. Jo resides in Central Florida with her husband and two daughters.